CHEMOTHER
COO

The Complete Guide to a Healthy Chemotherapy Diet: Recipes to Help You Through Your Treatment

REX LEWIS

Copyright © 2024 by REX LEWIS

All Rights Reserved.

Table of Contents

Introduction 5

CHAPTER ONE 12

  Synopsis of Chemotherapy 12

  Typical Side Effects 19

CHAPTER TWO 26

  Effect on Consumption of Nutrition 26

  The Value of a Balanced Diet 33

CHAPTER THREE 40

  Sustaining Body Mass and Weight 40

  Creating a Diet Friendly to Chemotherapy 46

CHAPTER FOUR 53

  Taking Care of Common Side Effects with Diet 53

  Meal Planning and Recipes 58

CHAPTER FIVE 66

Way of Life and Coping Mechanisms 66

How to Prevent and Treat Dehydration 74

Overcoming Obstacles and Maintaining Hope 81

In Summary 90

THE END 93

Introduction

Drugs are used in chemotherapy, a type of cancer treatment, to either kill or stop the growth of cancer cells. As a systemic treatment, the medications target certain healthy cells as well as the cancer cells by circulating throughout the body.

The following essential points can help you better understand chemotherapy:

1. Goal:

• **Destruction of Cancer Cells**: The main objective is to eradicate or stop the spread of cancer cells.

• **Systemic Treatment:** This approach targets cancer cells that may have spread outside of the original tumor by affecting the entire body.

2. Chemotherapy Types:

- **Combination therapy:** To maximize efficacy, several medications are frequently used together.

- **Adjuvant Therapy:** Used to get rid of any cancer cells that remained after radiation or surgery.

- **Neoadjuvant therapy**: used to reduce tumor size prior to surgery.

3. Administration:

- Oral or Intravenous (IV): Medications can be administered intravenously (IV) through a vein, orally as pills.

- Subcutaneous (SC) or intramuscular (IM): Certain medications are injected under the skin or into the muscle.

4. Frequency and Length:

- **Treatment Cycles:** Usually administered in cycles interspersed with rest intervals to facilitate the body's healing.

- **Frequency:** Depending on the particular regimen, this can be done every day, every week, or at various intervals.

5. Adverse Reactions:

- **Normal Cells Affected:** Bone marrow, digestive tract, and hair follicles are examples of healthy cells that might be impacted by fast growth.

- Typical side effects include anemia, decreased immunity, hair loss, nausea, fatigue, and appetite problems.

6. Handling Adverse Effects:

- **Supportive Care**: Medications and alterations to lifestyle to mitigate adverse effects.

- **Monitoring:** Frequent examinations and blood work to evaluate the effectiveness of treatment.

7. In Conjunction With Additional Therapies:

- **Surgery:** To remove tumors, surgery is frequently combined with other procedures.

- **Radiation therapy:** Used in conjunction to improve the efficacy of treatment.

8. Personalized Medicines:

- More recent medications target particular molecules implicated in the development of cancer.

- **Less Side Effects:** Targeted treatments try to do as little damage to healthy cells as possible.

9. Aftercare:

- **Observation:** Periodic reassessments to evaluate the reaction to therapy and handle any lingering consequences.

- **Survivorship Plans:** Emphasize preserving general health and averting relapses.

10. Support for Patients and Caregivers:

- **Emotional Support:** Handling the psychological and emotional effects of cancer treatment.

- **Support Groups:** Making connections with people who have gone through comparable circumstances.

Crucial Points to Remember:

- **Individual Variability:** Patients' reactions to chemotherapy might differ greatly from one another.

- **Personalized Treatment programs:** Based on the patient's preferences, general health, and the kind and stage of their cancer, oncologists customize treatment programs.

Open communication is crucial between patients receiving chemotherapy and their medical staff in order to resolve issues, control side effects, and guarantee the best results.

CHAPTER ONE
Synopsis of Chemotherapy

Drugs are used in chemotherapy, a type of cancer treatment, to either kill or stop the growth of cancer cells. As a systemic therapy, it affects both malignant and healthy cells by circulating throughout the body. Chemotherapy aims to reduce tumor size, stop cancer from spreading, and get rid of or manage cancer cells.

Essential Elements of Chemotherapy:

1. Classification of Drugs:

• **Cytotoxic Drugs:** They destroy cells, particularly cancer cells, that divide quickly.

- **Targeted therapies:** Medications that specifically target molecules implicated in the development of cancer.

- **Immunotherapy:** To combat cancer, it strengthens the immune system of the body.

2. Management:

- **Oral:** Medicine given orally in the form of pills or liquids.

- **Intravenous (IV):** injected straight into the circulation.

- **Subcutaneous (SC) or intramuscular (IM):** injected beneath the skin or into the muscle.

3. Therapy Objectives:

- **Curative:** Total eradication of malignant cells.

- **Palliative:** Reducing symptoms and enhancing life expectancy.

- **Adjuvant or Neoadjuvant:** Applied prior to or following radiation therapy or surgery.

4. Cycles of Treatment:

- **Cycles:** Treatments are usually given in cycles, with intervals of rest in between.

- **Frequency:** Relies on the kind and stage of the malignancy as well as the particular treatment regimen.

5. Adverse Reactions:

- **Normal Cell Impact:** Fast-growing, healthy cells are impacted.

- Typical side effects include anemia, decreased immunity, hair loss, fatigue, and nausea.

- Individual Variability: Patients may experience different side effects.

6. In conjunction with Additional Therapies:

- **Surgery:** Frequently performed either before or after to remove cancer cells that remain after a tumor has shrunk.

- **Radiation therapy:** Incorporated to improve the efficacy of treatment.

7. Observation and Modifications:

- **Routine Checkups:** Keeping an eye on how the patient is responding to therapy.

- **Modifications:** Depending on the patient's response and side effects, treatment plans may need to be adjusted.

8. Supportive Care: Medication: prescribed to control adverse reactions such as pain and nausea.

- **Lifestyle Modifications:** Stress reduction, exercise, and dietary changes.

9. Extended-Term Aspects:

• Follow-up Care: After treatment, routine examinations to keep an eye out for recurrences.

• Survival Plans: Stress the importance of general health and wellbeing.

10. Help for Patients:

• **Emotional Support:** Managing the psychological and emotional effects of cancer.

• **Support Groups:** Making connections with people experiencing comparable circumstances.

Obstacles & Things to Think About:

• **Side Effects:** Although supportive care might help manage side effects, chemotherapy frequently produces them.

- **Effect on Normal Cells:** Healthy cells that proliferate quickly, like those in the digestive system and bone marrow, may be impacted.

- **Individual Response:** Depending on the kind and stage of the cancer, different people respond differently to chemotherapy.

- **Developments:** Ongoing research results in the creation of novel medications and more specialized treatments.

Chemotherapy, in short, is an essential part of cancer treatment that tries to get rid of or manage cancer cells. Even while side effects can make chemotherapy difficult, advancements in supportive care and research help to improve results and patients' overall quality of life.

Typical Side Effects

Chemotherapy affects quickly dividing cells in both healthy and malignant cells, which can lead to a variety of side effects. Individual differences exist in the intensity and nature of side effects, which are contingent upon the pharmaceuticals used, their dosage, and the patient's general state of health. Here are some frequent side effects connected with chemotherapy:

1. Nausea and Vomiting:

- **Cause:** Irritation of the gastrointestinal tract.

- **Management:** Antiemetics, or anti-nausea drugs, may be recommended.

2. Fatigue:

- **Cause:** Causes a generalized weariness by affecting normal cells.

- **Management:** Sufficient sleep, healthy eating, and moderate exercise.

3. Alopecia, or Hair Loss:

Cause: Impacts hair follicle cells that divide quickly.

- **Management:** Hair usually grows back following therapy; wigs, scarves, or caps can be worn.

4. Anemia:

- **Cause:** Reduced red blood cell count, which results in weakness and exhaustion.

- **Management:** Red blood cell production-stimulating medications or blood transfusions.

- Neutropenia: A low white blood cell count that increases susceptibility to infections due to a decrease in white blood cells.

- **Management:** observation, application of growth stimulants, and, if required, administration of antibiotics.

6. Thrombocytopenia (Low Platelet Count):

- **Cause:** Platelets decrease, which raises the chance of bleeding.

- Management includes monitoring, platelet transfusions, and bleeding control measures.

7. Mucositis:

- **Cause:** Inflammation of the digestive tract and oral mucous membranes.

- **Management:** Mouthwash, good dental hygiene, and prescription drugs to reduce symptoms.

8. Peripheral neuropathy:

- **Cause:** Nerve damage resulting in pain, tingling, or numbness in the limbs.

- **Management:** Modifications to dosage, physical therapy, or medicine.

9. Modifications In Hunger:

- Cause: Modifications in flavor, nausea, or mouth sores can all impact hunger.

- **Management:** Meeting individual taste preferences and serving small, frequent meals.

10. Chemo Brain Cognitive Effects:

• Cause: Changes in memory and difficulty focusing.

• Management: Talking with medical professionals, getting enough sleep, and engaging in cognitive exercises.

11. Modifications to the Skin and Nails:

• **Origin:** Rashes, dry skin, or altered nail structure.

• **Handling:** Use moisturizers, stay away from strong washes, and keep your nails healthy.

12. A shift in appetite, metabolism, or fluid retention is the cause of weight changes.

- Management: When feasible, engage in exercise and a balanced diet.

Patients receiving chemotherapy must be transparent with their medical staff on any adverse effects they may be experiencing. During and after chemotherapy, supportive care interventions and treatment plan modifications can frequently assist control these side effects and enhance overall quality of life.

CHAPTER TWO
Effect on Consumption of Nutrition

The amount of nutrients taken and one's general nutritional state can both be significantly impacted by chemotherapy. Rapidly dividing cells are affected by the treatment, which affects healthy cells as well as cancerous ones, especially those found in the digestive tract. Chemotherapy might affect dietary intake in the following ways:

1. Nausea and Vomiting: Effect: Chemotherapy patients may have nausea and vomiting, which can make it difficult to eat and remain hydrated.

- **Management:** To treat these symptoms, doctors may prescribe anti-nausea drugs.

2. Appetite alterations: Impact: Chemotherapy may cause taste alterations, lack of appetite, or food aversions.

- **Management:** Patients are frequently instructed to emphasize short, frequent meals, select flavorless or bland foods, and drink plenty of water.

3. Mucositis:

- Impact: Eating might be uncomfortable due to tongue and throat inflammation.

- **Management:** It might be advised to eat cool, bland, and soft foods. Keeping your mouth clean is essential to avoiding infections.

4. Weight Changes:

- **Impact:** Depending on variables like hunger changes and metabolism changes, chemotherapy may cause weight gain or loss.

- **Management:** To maintain a healthy weight, dietary modifications, nutritional advice, and monitoring are crucial.

5. Anemia:

- **Effect:** Reduced oxygen delivery to tissues and weariness might arise from a decreased red blood cell count.

- **Management:** It may be advised to take iron supplements and eat meals high in iron.

6. Neutropenia:

- **Effect:** Low white blood cell count raises the possibility of illnesses, which makes it harder to eat particular foods.

- **Management:** It's crucial to handle food correctly, refrain from eating anything that's too raw or undercooked, and maintain appropriate hygiene.

7. Thrombocytopenia:

- **Effect:** Reduced platelet count might raise the chance of bleeding, which influences the selection and preparation of food.

- **Management:** Consume foods that are soft, easily chewed, and less likely to harm the mouth or digestive system.

8. Peripheral neuropathy:

- **Effect:** Hand and foot numbness, tingling, or pain might make it difficult to use cutlery and cook.

- **Management:** Using adaptive tools and making adjustments to food preparation methods may be beneficial.

9. Hydration:

- **Effect:** Dehydration can be exacerbated by nausea, vomiting, and taste alterations.

- **Management:** It's important for patients to drink enough fluids; they may need to try a variety of drinks to see what they tolerate.

10. Psychosocial Factors:

- **Impact:** Emotional and psychological elements like worry and stress can affect a person's appetite and eating preferences.

- **Management:** Involving a trained nutritionist, providing supportive care, and counseling can all help with these issues.

For those receiving chemotherapy, individualized nutritional treatment is crucial. Together with the medical staff, a trained dietician can design a plan that addresses the unique requirements and obstacles of the patient, with the goal of preserving sufficient nutrition and promoting general wellbeing both during and after chemotherapy.

The Value of a Balanced Diet

Sustaining a nutritious diet is essential for general health and becomes even more critical with different life stages and health issues, such as cancer and chemotherapy. The following are some main points emphasizing the significance of a nutritious diet:

1. Nutrient Support:

• Essential nutrients, including vitamins, minerals, proteins, carbs, and fats, are provided by a balanced diet and are necessary for the body to function properly.

• These nutrients are essential for the creation of energy generally, immune system support, and cellular function.

2. Assistance During Illness and Therapy: An appropriately balanced diet can assist in bolstering the body's resistance against the physical strain of ailments, such as cancer.

- The body may require more nutrition during chemotherapy, therefore maintaining strength and resilience can be aided by eating a good diet.

3. Function of the Immune System: Foods high in nutrients boost immunity, assisting the body in fending off infections and recuperating from sicknesses.

- This is especially crucial while receiving cancer treatment because chemotherapy might momentarily impair immunity.

4. Energy Levels: Consuming a nutritious diet gives you the energy you need to go about your everyday business and meet the physical demands of disease and treatment.

• Sustaining sufficient energy levels is crucial for effectively handling fatigue, a prevalent adverse reaction to chemotherapy.

5. Tissue Repair and Recovery: During and after chemotherapy, when the body may suffer cell damage, proteins, vital amino acids, and other nutrients are critical for tissue repair and recovery.

6. Weight Management: Eating well contributes to maintaining a healthy weight, which is critical for general health and can enhance the effectiveness of treatment.

• Maintaining a healthy weight helps lower the chance of problems and improve the body's capacity to withstand and react to medication.

7. Digestive Health: A diet high in fruits, vegetables, and fiber helps maintain digestive health by preventing constipation and encouraging regular bowel movements. This is crucial during cancer treatment because some chemotherapy medications can have an adverse effect on the digestive system.

8. Mental and Emotional Well-Being: Adequate diet can have a beneficial effect on one's mental and emotional health by giving one a sense of control and fostering optimism in the face of adversity.

• A healthy diet has been associated with improved mood, memory, and general quality of life.

9. Bone Health: To keep your bones healthy, you need to consume certain minerals including calcium and vitamin D.

• Chemotherapy and other cancer therapies can occasionally affect bone density, which emphasizes the importance of a healthy diet.

10. Reducing the Risk of Complications: An infection-prone diet can help lower the risk of nutritional deficiencies, infections, and a delayed recovery from cancer therapy.

Certain health issues, the type of cancer, and the stage of therapy can all affect an individual's nutritional requirements. It's critical that people receiving chemotherapy or other forms of cancer treatment collaborate with medical specialists, such as registered dietitians, to develop individualized nutrition programs that take into account their particular requirements and obstacles.

CHAPTER THREE
Sustaining Body Mass and Weight

Sustaining a healthy weight and muscular mass is especially crucial for those receiving chemotherapy or other forms of cancer treatment. Chemotherapy side effects, such as nausea, altered appetite, and exhaustion, might affect dietary intake and increase the risk of muscle atrophy and weight loss. During chemotherapy, the following techniques can help you maintain your weight and muscle mass:

1. A Diet Rich in Nutrients and Balanced:

• Eat a varied diet full of foods high in vital nutrients, such as fruits, vegetables, whole grains, lean meats, and healthy fats. Make sure your diet is well-balanced.

• Choose meals high in nutrients to get the most out of your vitamin and mineral intake without consuming too many calories.

2. Sufficient Consumption of Protein: Protein is necessary to preserve muscular mass. Eat a diet rich in lean meats, poultry, fish, eggs, dairy products, legumes, and nuts, among other high-protein foods.

• If necessary, take into account protein drinks or supplements under a doctor's supervision.

3. Regular Small Meals: It can be simpler to handle three big meals a day if you eat smaller, more often meals throughout the day. This can support consistent energy levels and help control nausea.

4. Hydration: Make sure you drink enough water because dehydration might make you feel tired. Clear broths, water, and herbal teas are healthy options. Refrain from consuming too much alcohol and coffee.

5. Managing Nausea: Assist your medical team in addressing nausea brought on by chemotherapy. It can be helpful to use anti-nausea drugs as directed and to change your diet to include more easily digested, bland meals.

6. Physical Activity: Take part in mild to moderate exercise, if tolerated. Exercise can enhance hunger, lessen weariness, and assist maintain muscular mass.

• Speak with your medical staff before beginning or altering any workout program.

7. Supplements: If consuming regular food isn't enough to meet calorie and nutrient requirements, think about taking nutritional supplements under the advice of a healthcare provider.

- If deficiencies are found, supplements containing vitamins and minerals might be advised.

8. High-Calorie Snacks: Include high-calorie snacks like cheese, yogurt, almonds, or smoothies with lots of protein in between meals.

- To get extra calories without consuming empty calories, pick nutrient-dense foods.

9. Meal Preparation and Preferences: Try a variety of meal preparation techniques to see which ones are the most agreeable and tolerable.

- Respect dietary needs and preferences while keeping nutritional objectives in mind.

10. Social Support and Counseling: Ask friends, relatives, or support groups for assistance. There is a connection between dietary intake and emotional health.

- For individualized advice and counseling, think about scheduling a consultation with a certified dietitian or nutritionist.

It's critical to remember that everyone has different nutritional requirements, and that creating a customized nutrition plan for chemotherapy requires the advice of medical professionals, particularly certified dietitians. Throughout the course of therapy, it may be required to conduct routine monitoring and make modifications to the plan in order to address evolving needs and adverse effects.

Creating a Diet Friendly to Chemotherapy

Creating a diet that is friendly to chemotherapy entails concentrating on nutrient-dense foods that offer vital vitamins, minerals, and energy while taking into account any side effects and difficulties associated with cancer treatment. The following are broad recommendations for designing a supporting diet during chemotherapy:

1. Highlight Foods Rich in Nutrients:

• **Fruits and Vegetables:** To guarantee a wide range of vitamins and antioxidants, select a choice of colorful fruits and vegetables. To make them easier to digest, steam or boil them.

• **Whole Grains:** For fiber and long-lasting energy, choose whole grains such brown rice, quinoa, oats, and whole wheat.

2. Lean Proteins: To maintain muscular mass, use lean protein sources including poultry, fish, and eggs. Salmon and other fish high in omega-3 fatty acids can be advantageous.

- Nuts and legumes: Include plant-based protein sources such nuts, lentils, and beans.

3. Healthy Fats: Add sources of healthy fats for energy and general wellbeing, such as avocado, nuts, and olive oil. It can be simpler to digest these lipids.

- **Fatty Fish:** Fish high in omega-3 fatty acids, such as salmon, helps reduce inflammation.

4. Hydration: To avoid dehydration, drink plenty of water and herbal teas. Clear broths, water, and herbal teas are healthy options. Limit your alcohol and caffeine intake.

5. Frequently Eat Smaller Meals: To control nausea and save energy, eat smaller, more frequent meals throughout the day.

6. Simple to Chew and Digest Foods: Select foods that are prepared, soft, and simple to chew and digest. Vegetable steaming, stews, and soups can all be easy on the stomach.

7. High-Calorie Snacks:

- Incorporate high-calorie snacks, including cheese, nuts, or smoothies that are packed with nutrients, in between meals.

8. Protein Supplements: To support protein consumption, if necessary, think about using protein smoothies or supplements.

9. Handling Nausea:

- **Ginger:** Include ginger in your diet as it has the potential to reduce nausea.

- **Boring Foods:** When experiencing nausea, choose non-greasy, bland foods.

10. Tracking Blood Counts:

- **Iron-Rich Diet:** Consume foods high in iron to promote the synthesis of red blood cells.

- **Vitamin C:** Iron-rich diets and vitamin C-rich foods work together to improve iron absorption.

11. Easy-to-Chew Options: • If you have trouble chewing, go for softer foods like purees, smoothies, or cooked grains.

12. Social Support and Counseling: Seek out assistance from loved ones, friends, or support groups. For individualized advice, think about contacting a qualified dietitian or nutritionist.

13. Reduce Your Intake of Processed and Sugary Foods: Reduce your consumption of processed and sugary foods because they have little nutritional value and may cause inflammation.

14. Individual Preferences:

• Respect one's own dietary needs and desires while staying within the parameters of dietary objectives.

Keep in mind that every person reacts differently to food, so it's critical to pay attention to your body and modify as needed. Speaking with a member of your healthcare team, such as a qualified dietician, can assist customize food recommendations to your unique situation and take care of any issues or difficulties you may have while undergoing chemotherapy.

CHAPTER FOUR
Taking Care of Common Side Effects with Diet

Making certain dietary choices to improve general well-being and assist control symptoms is part of managing typical side effects of chemotherapy with diet. The following dietary approaches can help with frequent adverse effects of chemotherapy:

1. Queasy and Regurgitating:

• **Ginger:** Add some ginger to your meals. Nausea may be reduced by consuming ginger tea, ginger candies, or fresh ginger added to food.

• **Boring Foods:** Go for foods that are simple to digest, such rice, crackers, or boiled potatoes.

- **Smaller, More Often Meals:** Avoid having an empty stomach, which can exacerbate nausea, by eating smaller, more frequent meals.

2. Modifications in Appetite:

- **High-Calorie Snacks:** To increase calorie intake, include high-nutrient snacks like cheese, almonds, or smoothies in between meals.

- **Regular, Small Meals:** It might be simpler to handle eating smaller meals more frequently.

3. Mucositis and Mouth Sores:

- **Soft, Easy-to-Chew Foods:** To reduce inflammation, choose for prepared, soft, and easily chewable foods.

- **Steer away of Spicy or Acidic Foods:** These foods have the potential to exacerbate mouth sores.

- **Mild Mouth Rinses:** Use a warm water and baking soda or salt mixture to gently rinse your mouth.

4. Fatigue:

- Maintain a well-balanced diet consisting of a combination of healthy fats, proteins, and carbohydrates to provide long-lasting energy.

- **Fluids:** Maintain adequate fluids since weariness can be exacerbated by dehydration.

5. Iron-Rich Foods: Consume foods high in iron, such as dark leafy greens, beans, lentils, and lean meats.

- **Vitamin C:** Iron-rich diets and vitamin C-rich foods work together to improve iron absorption.

6. Constipation: Eat High-Fiber meals: Consume whole grains, fruits, vegetables, legumes, and other high-fiber meals.

- **Hydration:** To assist ease constipation, consume lots of water.

7. Diarrhea:

- **BRAT Diet:** To help harden stools, think about include bananas, rice, applesauce, and toast into your diet.

- **Steer Clear of Trigger items:** Be aware of and steer clear of items like caffeine and spicy foods that can cause diarrhea.

8. Peripheral Neuropathy: B-Vitamin-rich foods, such as leafy greens, almonds, and whole grains, can help maintain the health of your nerves.

- **Omega-3 Fatty Acids:** Flaxseeds and fatty fish may have anti-inflammatory properties.

9. Taste Modifications:

- **Taste-Test Flavors:** Vary herbs and spices to bring forth taste notes.

- **Foods at Room or Cold Temperatures:** Foods at these temperatures may have milder smells and scents.

It's important to remember that everyone reacts differently to different things, so figuring out what works best for you may require some trial and error. Speaking with a member of your healthcare team, such as a qualified dietician, can also help with specific concerns you may have about your chemotherapy treatment and offer individualized assistance.

Meal Planning and Recipes

Meal planning during chemotherapy involves creating nutritious and easily digestible meals that address potential side effects and support overall well-being. Here are some general tips for meal planning, along with a few recipes tailored to common side effects:

Tips for Meal Planning:

- **Smaller, More Often Meals**: To control nausea and preserve energy, choose for smaller, more frequent meals.

- **Balanced Nutrients:** For long-lasting energy, make sure that each meal has an appropriate amount of healthy fats, proteins, and carbs.

- Maintain adequate hydration. As part of your daily fluid intake, include clear broths, herbal teas, and water.

Simple Foods to Digestion:

When choosing foods to prevent irritation for people with mouth sores, choose for soft, prepared, and easily chewed items.

- **Gentle Cooking Techniques:** To make food easier to digest, use gentle cooking techniques like steaming, boiling, or baking.

- **Nutrient-Dense Snacks:** Include high-nutrient snacks like smoothies, yogurt, and almonds in your diet in between meals.

- **Avoid Strong Odors:** If you're easily offended by fragrances, stay away from foods with strong aromas and go for cold or room temperature instead.

- **Try Different Flavors:** For people who are experiencing taste alterations, try different herbs and spices to enhance flavors.

Sample Cookbooks:

1. Chicken Soup with Ginger and Lemon:

Ingredients:

- Skinny, boneless chicken breast
- sodium-free chicken broth
- chopped carrots, fresh ginger, and slices
- Quinoa or rice
- Juice from lemons
- chopped fresh parsley

Guidelines:

- Put the chicken breast, carrots, ginger, and chicken stock in a saucepan. Simmer until the chicken is tender.
- Once the chicken is shredded, add the rice or quinoa and simmer until the grains are tender.
- Before serving, stir in lemon juice and fresh parsley.

2. Mashed Sweet Potatoes:

Ingredients:

- Diced and peeled sweet potatoes
- Olive oil or butter
- Optional: nutmeg or cinnamon

Instructions:

1. Steam or boil sweet potatoes until they are soft. Season with salt and pepper to taste.
2. Blend using butter or olive oil, and if preferred, sprinkle with cinnamon or nutmeg.
3. Add pepper and salt for seasoning.

3. Cooked Quinoa With Vegetables In A Stir-Fry:

Ingredients

- mixed veggies, including carrots, broccoli, and bell peppers
- Diced chicken or tofu
- Soy sauce

- minced ginger and garlic
- oil from sesame

Directions:

1. Sauté the ginger and garlic in sesame oil in a skillet.
2. Cook the diced chicken or tofu by stirring it in.
3. Add the cooked quinoa and mixed vegetables. Add a drizzle of soy sauce and mix thoroughly.

- Ingredients for the fourth fruit smoothie: mixed berries (strawberries, blueberries, raspberries)
  - Banana

- Plant-based yogurt or Greek yogurt
- Honey is optional.
- Cubes of ice

- **Directions:** Blend banana, yogurt, ice cubes, and berries until smooth.

- If desired, add honey. To adjust consistency, add milk or water.

Remember to adapt recipes based on individual preferences and dietary restrictions. It's essential to consult with healthcare professionals, including a registered dietitian, for personalized meal planning that suits your specific needs during chemotherapy.

CHAPTER FIVE
Way of Life and Coping Mechanisms

A supportive network and lifestyle modifications are crucial for minimizing the negative effects of chemotherapy and helping patients cope. The following are some essential lifestyle and helpful tactics:

1. Keep Lines of Communication Open:

• **With Your Healthcare Team:** Share your symptoms, worries, and any potential side effects with your healthcare team.

• **With Loved Ones:** Establish a solid support network by communicating your needs and feelings to family and friends.

2. A Balanced Lifestyle:

- **Rest and Sleep:** To support general wellbeing, make sure you receive enough sleep and give it priority.

- **Physical Activity:** Take part in mild to moderate exercise on a tolerated basis. See your medical team before beginning or altering an exercise program.

3. Tension Management: To reduce tension and anxiety, engage in deep breathing exercises, mindfulness training, or meditation.

- **Support Services:** For mental health, consider therapy, counseling, or support groups.

4. Nutritional Assistance:

- **Speak with a Dietitian:** Create a customized nutrition plan with the help of a trained dietitian that takes into account your particular requirements and obstacles.

- **Remain Hydrated:** To promote general health, stay well hydrated, particularly during therapy.

5. Holistic Therapies:

- **Acupuncture or Massage:** Complementary therapies like acupuncture or massage can help some people get better from side effects including exhaustion and nausea.

• **Yoga or Tai Chi:** Mild workouts like these can increase flexibility, lower stress levels, and promote general wellbeing.

6. Adequate Support for Adverse Reactions:

• **Medication:** To control side effects including pain or nausea, use prescribed drugs as instructed.

• **Topical Creams:** Use suggested ointments or creams for side effects pertaining to the skin.

7. Adaptive Strategies:

- **Assistive equipment**: To improve safety and independence, think about utilizing assistive equipment if you're having trouble moving around or coordinating.

- **Adaptive Clothes**: Opt for relaxed-fitting, comfy attire that can adapt to any physical shifts.

8. Mind-Body Connection:

- **Creative Expression:** To express feelings and foster a sense of control, partake in creative endeavors like writing, music, or painting.

- **Visualization or Guided Imagery:** When facing difficult situations, concentrate on positive imagery by using visualization techniques.

9. Social Support:

- **Friends and Family:** Encircle yourself with a network of friends and family that are there to support you and who can offer both practical and emotional help.

- **Support Groups:** Get in touch with people going through similar experiences by joining a support group for cancer patients.

10. Frequent Exams and Observations:

- **Follow-up Appointments:** Keep track of treatment progress and address any issues by attending routine check-ups.

• **Blood Tests:** Maintain the schedule of required blood tests to evaluate general health and response to treatment.

11. Modifications at Home:

• Create a Comfortable Ambience: Make your house cozy and favorable to unwinding.

• **Make Assistance Arrangements:** Be prepared for unforeseen difficulties and make arrangements for help with everyday duties as needed.

12. Advocacy and Education:

- Remain Informed: Become knowledgeable about your illness, available treatments, and any possible adverse effects.

- **Speak Up for Yourself:** Ask questions and get information from your healthcare team to help you be an active advocate for your own health.

Recall that every person's experience with chemotherapy is different. Customize these tactics to your own requirements and inclinations, and don't be afraid to ask for help and advice from experts. Throughout your cancer experience, your healthcare team—which includes nurses, oncologists, and support services—can offer invaluable assistance.

How to Prevent and Treat Dehydration

Maintaining adequate hydration is essential during chemotherapy, since it promotes general health and aids in the management of possible adverse effects. Chemotherapy-related side effects such as nausea, vomiting, diarrhea, or altered taste buds can occasionally result in dehydration. The following advice will help you remain hydrated and prevent dehydration while receiving chemotherapy:

Advice on Maintaining Hydration:

1. Regular Water Consumption:

• Sip water continuously all day long. If you find it difficult to down bigger portions all at once, sip little amounts.

• Keep an easily accessible reusable water bottle with you to help you stay hydrated.

2. Hydrating Foods:

• Include foods high in water in your diet, such oranges, cucumbers, and watermelon, among other fruits and vegetables.

• Broths and soups also increase dietary intake of nutrients and liquids.

3. Herbal Teas and Infusions: To add diversity to your fluid intake, choose for herbal teas or infusions that are free of caffeine.

• Limit your intake of caffeinated drinks because they can cause dehydration.

4. Electrolyte-Rich liquids:

• If you're feeling queasy or have diarrhea, give electrolyte-rich liquids some thought.

• Homemade electrolyte beverages or commercial oral rehydration solutions can assist restore electrolytes that have been lost.

5. Coconut Water: This naturally occurring electrolyte source can also serve as a hydrating substitute.

6. Establish Hydration Goals: Determine your daily water consumption target by taking into account your unique requirements. Your medical staff is qualified to offer advice.

Controlling Sweating:

1. Identify the Symptoms of Dehydration: Common symptoms include dark urine, lightheadedness, fast heartbeat, parched lips, and reduced urination.

- Let your medical team know if you continue to feel the effects of dehydration.

2. Handle Nausea and Vomiting:

- As these symptoms might lead to dehydration, collaborate with your medical team to manage nausea and vomiting brought on by chemotherapy.

- Anti-nausea drugs could be recommended to assist manage these adverse effects.

3. Track Fluid Loss: If you have diarrhea, keep an eye on your fluid intake and get help if it doesn't go away.

- Inform your medical staff of any changes in your bowel habits.

4. Replenish Electrolytes: If electrolyte imbalance coexists with dehydration, think about ingesting meals or beverages that contain electrolytes, like oral rehydration solutions or sports drinks.

5. Hydration throughout Treatment: To support your body's reaction to treatment, drink plenty of water before to, during, and after chemotherapy treatments.

6. Speak with Your Healthcare Team: Seek advice and potential interventions from your healthcare team as soon as dehydration becomes a problem.

- Intravenous (IV) fluids may be required in extreme situations.

7. Modify Diet for Comfort: When suffering symptoms like nausea or taste changes, modify your diet to include items that are more tolerable.

8. Maintain Regular Check-ups: Schedule routine examinations with your medical team to keep an eye on your general health and to handle any new issues that may arise.

It's critical to customize your hydration plan to your unique requirements and tastes. Speaking with a qualified dietitian and other members of your healthcare team about any unique issues you may be experiencing with staying hydrated throughout chemotherapy will help you receive individualized advice and support.

Overcoming Obstacles and Maintaining Hope

It might be difficult to overcome obstacles and keep a cheerful attitude during chemotherapy, but doing so is essential for the general wellbeing of those receiving treatment. The following techniques can assist in overcoming obstacles and cultivating an optimistic outlook:

1. Establish a Robust Support System:

• Encircle yourself with a network of friends, family, and medical professionals who will support you.

• Talk to loved ones about your thoughts and feelings, and ask for support and consolation.

2. Remain Informed:

• Become knowledgeable about your illness, the course of therapy, and any possible adverse effects. Anxiety might be reduced by comprehending the procedure.

• Be open and honest in your communication with your healthcare staff.

3. Have Reasonable Expectations:

• Recognize that there may be difficulties associated with chemotherapy, and it's acceptable to acknowledge both the good and bad times.

• Throughout treatment, have reasonable expectations for both your abilities and yourself.

4. Concentrate on What You Can Control:

• Determine which areas of your life you have control over, then give those your attention. This could entail making decisions regarding your daily schedule, workout regimen, and food.

- Assume responsibility for your own care to empower yourself.

5. Employ relaxation and mindfulness techniques:

- To relieve tension and encourage relaxation, try mindfulness exercises, deep breathing, meditation, or guided imagery.

- Take into account enrolling in a yoga or meditation session designed specifically for those receiving therapy.

6. Celebrate Little Victories:

- Throughout your therapeutic journey, recognize and commemorate your little victories.

- Take pleasure in small victories and instances of resiliency.

7. Creative Expression: Use artistic, musical, or literary endeavors as a way to express yourself. Moreover, using creative outlets as a coping mechanism for emotions can be helpful.

8. Seek Professional Support: To deal with emotional difficulties, think about speaking with a therapist, counselor, or joining a support group.

- Expert assistance can offer direction on coping mechanisms and psychological health.

9. Keep Up a Healthy Lifestyle: To promote both physical and mental health, concentrate on eating a balanced diet, exercising frequently (as tolerated), and getting enough sleep.

- Seek advice from medical professionals for tailored lifestyle suggestions.

10. Remain in Touch: '

- Maintain communication, even if it's only virtually, with loved ones. Emotional support can be obtained through social ties.

- Talk about your experiences with people who could be facing comparable difficulties.

11. Gratitude Practice:

- Develop a gratitude practice by thinking back on all of the good things in your life, no matter how little.

- Gratitude can improve a good outlook and help divert attention from difficulties.

12. Remain Adaptable and Flexible:

- Acknowledge that unforeseen difficulties can occur and that plans would need to be modified.

- Remain adaptable and willing to change course as necessary.

13. Honor Self-Care:

- Give top priority to self-care pursuits that offer solace and calm, including reading, having a warm bath, or going outside.

14. Keep Your Sense of Humor:

- Look for humor and levity in everyday situations. Laughing is a great coping mechanism when faced with hardship.

15. Express Your Feelings:

- Give yourself permission to communicate a variety of feelings, such as anger, fear, or grief. Writing in a journal or speaking with a reliable friend can be healing.

Recall that each person's journey is distinct, and it's acceptable to ask for assistance when required. Having a positive outlook does not imply disregarding difficulties; rather, it means overcoming them with resiliency and hope. Do not be reluctant to seek further assistance from mental health specialists if symptoms of distress continue.

In Summary

In conclusion, receiving chemotherapy can be very difficult on a physical and mental level. However, people can travel through this path with resiliency and hope if they have the correct plans in place and support networks. Prioritizing self-care, keeping lines of communication open with medical providers, and relying on family support are crucial.

• During chemotherapy, patients can cultivate a positive outlook and sense of control by learning about available treatment options, engaging in mindfulness and relaxation practices, and keeping an eye out for tiny successes along the journey. Adopting a healthy lifestyle that includes frequent exercise, wholesome food, and enough sleep can also improve general wellbeing and the body's capacity to tolerate therapy.

• Through all of the challenges, there are times during the chemotherapy journey when you can feel joy, thankfulness, and connection. In times of hardship, finding moments of fun and camaraderie, expressing creativity, and celebrating achievements can all help people become stronger and more resilient.

In the end, each person's experience with chemotherapy is distinct, and it's critical to respect one's own feelings and experiences during the process.

People can go through chemotherapy with grace and resolve, coming out stronger on the other side, if they embrace the trials with courage and keep an optimistic outlook.

THE END

Printed in Great Britain
by Amazon